The Good Bladder Guide

For Women

A D-I-Y Guide to Solving Bladder Problems

Jacqueline Hearn
MSc RGN RHV

Contents

Introduction

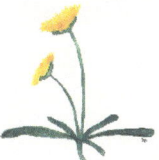

Is your bladder behaving badly? Having problems is one of the most embarrassing but unnecessary ailments we women have to suffer. One in five women experience damp knickers at least once a week. Getting up in the night, worries when coughing or sneezing, frequency, and not quite making the loo in time are all very common problems that can be rectified. Seeking professional help can seem daunting and embarrassing. Information and advice is hard to find.

However, self-help success rates for totally solving these problems are incredibly high. Medical interventions are very rarely needed.

This DIY guide will enable you to re-establish who is in charge here – you or your bladder!

No medical interventions. No gadgets. Just help to find out why you have the problem and clear guidelines to follow to solve the problem.

You will see a dramatic improvement within two months.

Starting with refreshing your knowledge of normal bladder function, the book enables you to define your individual problem. Simple, clear instructions will guide you and help you chart your improvement. The instructions are safe and non-invasive.

This is a book about bladder problems for women, so I have only just mentioned men's problems and bowel problems. There is also a glossary of medical terms.

Good Luck!

Golden Rules for a Good Bladder

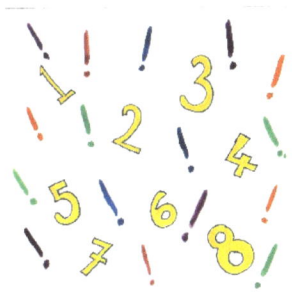

Be in charge of your bladder. Don't let it be in charge of you.

Drink at least two litres of fluid every day.

Pass 200-400 mls of urine at each visit.

Do not consume large amounts of tea, coffee or alcohol.

Do Pelvic Floor Exercises every day, but **every hour** if you have a bladder problem.

Pass urine about ten times a day.

Do not get up at night to pass urine. Well, only occasionally!

Make sure that you are not constipated.

Solving Your Bladder Problem

Toilet-visiting patterns are the result of years of training so that they fit in with our lifestyle. Everyone's patterns are unique, and problems occur when the bladder is in charge of our lifestyle rather than the reverse.

Problems as diverse as visiting the loo every half an hour to having to wear pads because of accidental passing of urine can be solved. Please do not expect overnight cures, as the timescale before any significant improvement is seen may be two months or more.

Start with doing Pelvic Floor Exercises NOW and every waking hour for the foreseeable future. Then, find a spare couple of days to fill out the 24-hour chart at the back of the book to find out what is happening between you and your bladder.

With the knowledge required, you will then be able to follow the guidelines and put into action a plan that will give you a well-behaved bladder that you can take anywhere. It sounds easy but it will take time and perseverance.

A good, basic knowledge of what is happening and what should be happening in the process of making and passing urine, a few tricks and a couple of months of intensive practice will see the problem of inappropriate passing of urine disappear.

The Process of Making and Passing Urine

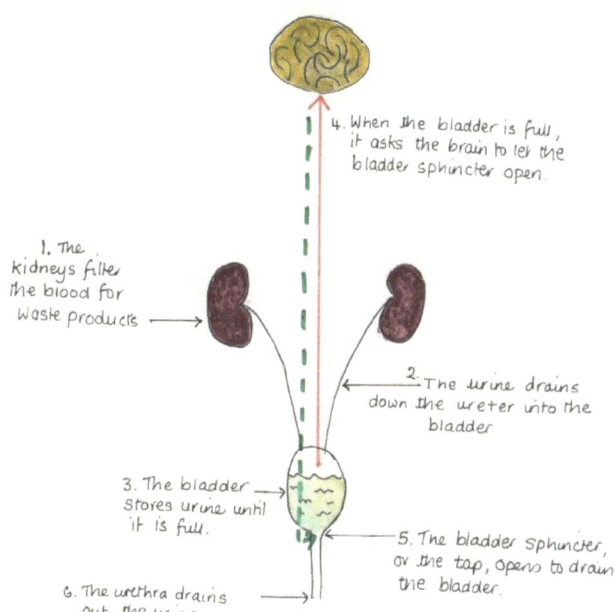

4. When the bladder is full, it asks the brain to let the bladder sphincter open.

1. The kidneys filter the blood for waste products →

2. The urine drains down the ureter into the bladder

3. The bladder stores urine until it is full. →

5. The bladder sphincter, or the tap, opens to drain the bladder.

6. The urethra drains out the urine →

Everyone's bladder habits are individual, but it is useful to know what is in the realms of normal. It is also useful to know the basic mechanics.

The kidneys continually sieve the blood for waste products. This waste is called urine. Although the kidneys are working all the time they do tend to slow down dramatically at night when we are asleep. About same amount of waste will be filtered but with much less fluid so this is why you expect your urine to be dark and concentrated in the mornings.

Urine is transported from the kidneys via the two ureters to the bladder where it is stored. The bladder has similar properties to a balloon. It deflates when empty and can expand as necessary to fill up with urine.

When the bladder is nearly full, a message is sent from the bladder, via the nervous system, to the brain. The brain then waits until a convenient time, say when a toilet is available, and then sends another message back down the nervous system to tell the bladder sphincter, which is rather like a tap, that it is now all right to open and pass urine.

In a baby, there is no choice in timing of passing urine as the messages to and from the brain are not mature, so once the bladder is full, the sphincter opens and urine is passed. But once the brain/bladder pathway has matured and toilet training has commenced the choice of when to spend a penny is then available.

Habit and circumstance will mould our own unique patterns of passing urine.

We expect to pass urine about ten times a day, every two to three hours, but usually more frequently in the morning.

Our urine should be much stronger on the first morning visit as the kidneys have been asleep and the resultant high concentration of waste products needs to be filtered.

We should not have to get up in the night to pass urine.

We should decide, within a reasonable time, when we want to pass urine, even if our bladder is full.

A Typical Normal 24- hour Urine Chart				
Time	Volume Of urine	Damp or Change of pad	Reason for dampness	Other notes
07.30	650 mls			
08.15	200mls			
09.00	200mls			
11.15	350mls			
14.45	300mls			
15.45	400mls			
17.45	350mls			
20.30	300mls			
23.00	300mls			
Total	2850 mls			No dampness. No problems

So what can alter these simple processes?

*Be aware that you can have more than
one problem!*

Kidney related Problems

The kidneys should just tick-over at night. To all events and purposes, they should go to sleep unless encouraged to stay awake. However, they can be wide-awake even though we are asleep, and if they do stay awake, they produce the same amount of fluid each hour as they do during the daytime. Obviously, the result will be a need to wake up to empty the bladder.

The amount of waste products sieved by the kidneys remains constant throughout the 24-hour period so our first morning visit should contain quite dark urine because the same amount of waste is in a smaller amount of fluid.

If you do have to pass urine during the night, it may be the result of tea, coffee or alcohol being ingested too late in the evening. These products are called "diuretics", which are substances that make the kidneys filter more fluid with the waste products.

Stress may be another reason for the kidneys not being able to settle down for a good night's rest. If the body is on heightened awareness for any reason then all the organs will remain ready for action. The kidneys, therefore, carry on producing daytime amounts of urine.

Another and the most usual cause for having to pass urine at night is habit. When you wake up in the night, as we all do, but then feel that you might as well empty your bladder, the trip to the loo will wake up the kidneys and produce more urine than normal. Over months this may well become a more than a once a night habit. Unless you feel that your bladder is really full, it is a good idea to resist the trip to the loo, turn over and go back to sleep.

Bladder related Problems

Once urine is excreted by the kidneys, it is taken by the ureters to the bladder. The pelvic floor muscles support the bladder. The bladder works well as a container if your urine isn't too strong, you are not constipated, and you have good pelvic floor muscles.

If you are constipated, your bowel may press on your bladder giving you false messages as to if and when you need to pass urine.

The bladder does not like strong urine. It irritates the wall of the bladder, and makes you want to pass urine more frequently. Many people with urinary problems drink less fluid to try and help stave-off the problems, but it, unfortunately, accentuates the problem. Drinking at least two litres of alcohol/caffeine free liquid is advised daily.

Many people pass urine too frequently! Passing urine too frequently is also not good for the bladder. The bladder needs to practice holding a reasonable amount of urine, and passing urine hourly is not helping this. Little and often can be caused by cystitis, an infection in the bladder, where a burning sensation is felt when passing urine. If frequency occurs without a burning sensation then the problem may well be down to habit.

The bladder sphincter is like a tap turning on the flow of urine, and it needs the support of good pelvic floor muscles. It needs the support of good, clear messages from the brain to tell it when it is convenient to pass urine ensuring that we are in charge, not our bladders.

Being in control of the bladder sphincter is rather like challenging the school bully in the playground. Once you're back in charge, you'll wonder what the problem was, but presently it may seem too big to handle.

If your pelvic floor muscles are in poor shape then both the bladder and bladder sphincter will not be supported enough when extra strain is put upon them. This may happen when we sneeze, cough, or exercise. The result will be an inability to prevent a leakage of urine.

Pelvic Floor Exercises

The pelvic floor muscles are like a trampoline. They should support the bladder and the tube that we pass urine through, the urethra. When we pass urine, our bladders tighten and our pelvic floor muscles relax. Once we finish passing urine, the pelvic floor muscles should then tighten back up. Childbirth definitely weakens these muscles, and so does getting older. However, we can easily get them back into check, and here is how.

Tighten the muscle in your vagina, as if trying to stop spending a penny, drawing upwards, and hold for about three seconds. Then relax the muscle. Repeat five times, relaxing the muscle in between. To check you have the correct muscle, you can insert a finger into your vagina whilst tightening the muscle. You should feel it tighten.

Try not to tighten the muscles in your buttocks, thighs or abdomen whilst doing the exercises.

Do not do the exercises with a full bladder. **Never** try to stop spending a penny midway through a flow of urine. Either of these can actually further weaken the pelvic floor.

During the next few days gradually increase the exercises until you are doing ten, holding each for three seconds, every hour.

Doing Pelvic Floor Exercises, PFEs, ten times each hour will, undoubtedly, improve the function of your bladder sphincter. This is because the sphincter will not be carrying the strain of holding the weight of a full bladder.

The pelvic floor will be holding the weight, and regaining its old job.

NB. As other people will not be aware of you doing these exercises, you can do them anywhere. However, as we are all human, it is difficult to keep doing something day-in day-out with no positive feedback for, say, two or more months.

I have tried a few ways of making sure I do PFEs every hour, and the only way that works for me is to tick off each time I do them on a daily chart. The chart has to be in view so that I remind myself when the next ten exercises are due.

What is Happening to You?

To be able to alleviate your bladder problem, you need to know clearly what is happening to you during a twenty-four hour period.

I suggest that, over a period of a couple of days, perhaps a weekend, use a plastic measuring jug to measure your urine each time you go. Measure the amount and frequency of visits. Record any dampness or downright accidents. Record any reasons that leakage occurs, for example, sneezing, coughing or running. You'll find charts in the back of this book.

The chart will enable you to diagnose your bladder problem or problems and provide the necessary solutions to put you back in charge.

Please remember that it is necessary that you are drinking at least two litres of fluid over and above drinks of tea, coffee and alcohol.
Tea, coffee and alcohol are diuretics. They encourage the kidneys to filter out more fluid than they should and this will result in the body being a little dehydrated.

Once you have completed the chart compare the answers given in the following chapters. You may well have some problems in more than one category.

Frequency

This is a debilitating condition that may have worsened insidiously over the years. Searching out public toilets and dreading long car journeys have become second nature. Be sure to follow the advice and you should see a significant improvement within a couple of months.

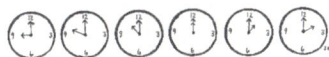

Stress Incontinence

Damp pants or even worst when you sneeze, cough or laugh is very embarrassing. Wearing pads make you worry if you may smell a little. Your urine may be very strong as you have been tackling the problem by trying to make less urine. Nothing seems to work. You will be so pleased and surprised by the improvement once you have been doing pelvic floor exercises. Redo the chart monthly to provide proof that you are improving.

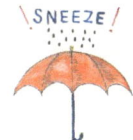

Urge Incontinence

Commencing the flow of urine too early can be very exasperating. You may have held on to go for quite a long time but when you are nearly in the loo you start to go. Your brain is alerting your bladder sphincter prematurely. Help is available.

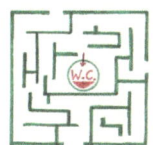

Getting Up at Night to Pass Urine

It is unnecessary to pass urine at night. It can become an undesirable habit   increasing to two or even three times a night. How tiring! Start sleeping through the night very soon.

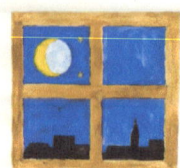

Cystitis

Ouch! If you suffer from cystitis you may well have been cutting down on fluids and making it worst. A doctor's visit will be necessary but prevention is in your court.

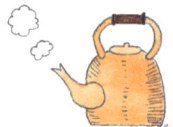

Male Incontinence

Women are more likely to suffer from bladder problems than men. Childbirth weakens the pelvic floor and the result may be stress bladder problems. Other bladder problems are found in both men and women and the solutions will be the same. Men may have prostate problems and a GP visit is advised.

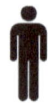

Passing Urine Frequently

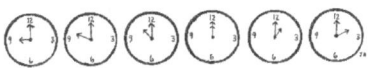

A Typical 24-hour Urine Chart Showing Frequency				
Time	Volume of urine	Damp or Change of pad	Reason for dampness	Other notes
07.30	300mls			
08.30	150 mls			
09.30	100mls			
10.00	50mls			Had to go before I went out
10.45	100mls			
11.30	100mls			
12.45	100mls			
13.45	100mls			
15.00	100mls			
16.30	150mls			
18.00	100mls			
19.30	100mls			
21.00	100mls			
23.00	50mls			
Total	1600mls			

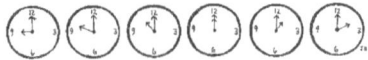

Passing Urine Frequently

If the chart shows that you are passing urine every hour or more and pass 150mls or less each time, you have 'frequency' which, I don't need to tell you, makes you a slave to your bladder. Whenever you go out, you have to spy out the toilets, and long journeys are a nightmare.

Even though it is hard to believe, your bladder will have the capacity to hold more urine. It is a balloon-like vessel. However, you need to gradually let it stretch to hold more, and for you to get used to the feeling comfortable having a fuller bladder.

1. Make sure that you are drinking at least two litres of fluid each day so that your urine isn't too strong and being an irritant on the wall of the bladder. You may well have cut down drastically to try to improve your lifestyle but this would have had the opposite effect.

2. Do your PFEs hourly so that your pelvic floor can easily hold an enlarged capacity.

3. Reduce the amount of tea, coffee and alcohol for a while so that your brain can get clear messages from your bladder.

4. For the next two weeks, try to last 15 minutes' longer than you want to before each time you pass urine. Divert your thoughts perhaps by reading a chapter of a good book, or other thought-provoking activity.

5. Repeat the chart after two weeks and see if there is any increase in volume of urine passed. You should see an increase. Encourage yourself to keep increasing the intervals between passing urine until you reach intervals of at least a couple of hours and pass between 250 and 400mls each time.

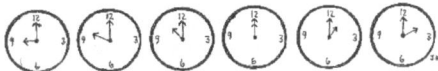

Stress Incontinence

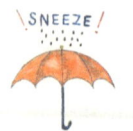

Time	Volume of urine	Damp or Change of pad	Reason for dampness	Other notes
		A Typical 24-hour Urine Chart Stress Incontinence		
07.30	500mls	No		Urine very strong
08.15	150mls	No		
09.00	100mls	Change of damp pad	Running for the bus	
10.30	200mls	No		
12.00	150mls	Change of damp pad	Sneezing whilst standing at photocopier	
14.00	200mls	No		
16.00	150 mls	No	Had to go to the loo as I felt a little smelly, but pad was dry so no problem	
17.30	150mls	No	Went to loo just before catching the bus home	
18.15	50mls	Soaked pad	Very tired from work. Walked quickly home	
22.00	100mls			
Total	1750mls			

Stress Incontinence

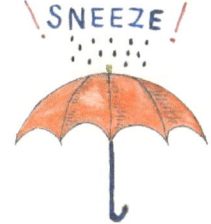

If the chart shows that you are leaking a little, or sometimes a lot, of urine when you cough, sneeze, run or perform similar activities, you have "stress incontinence'. Please be assured that however bad it is, it is not a permanent feature of your life.

1. The good news is that your problem is the most straightforward one to solve. I'm afraid it's those PFEs, though, and you won't see any appreciable difference for a good couple of months. How are you going to keep them up hourly every day? Please do them 10 times every hour. Get encouragement from anywhere you can. Bribe yourself, applaud yourself, cover your house with 'post-its'! I find that I do need to physically tick them off on a chart every hour, a chart that is in constant view.

2. You may have decreased your intake of fluid to counter the embarrassing dampness. Your urine will therefore be quite strong and therefore an irritant. Cut down on tea, coffee

and alcohol, and make sure you drink at least two litres of fluid a day. This will improve the clarity of messages from your bladder to your brain.

3. Repeat the chart after a month and you should see that there are fewer accidents, but keep up the regime and you will see that within six months there will be no more accidents. Honestly!

The day that you no longer need to wear pads is in sight. Keep up the exercises!

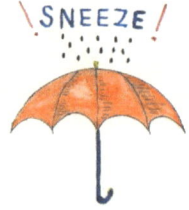

Urge Incontinence

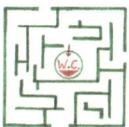

A Typical 24 Hour Urine Chart Urge Incontinence				
Time	Volume Of urine	Damp or Change of pad	Reason for dampness	Other notes
07.30	500mls			
08.30	200mls			
09.30	200mls			
11.30	250mls	Damp	Had to wait in queue in Ladies' Loo	
13.00	300mls			
14.00	100mls			Went to loo because I was thinking about it.
17.30	300mls	Damp	Another queue in the Ladies	
19.00	150mls	Very damp pad	Felt I needed to go whilst in the shop but waited until I got home. Started going as I got into the bathroom	
21.00	200mls			
23.00	100mls			
Total	2250 mls			

Urge Incontinence

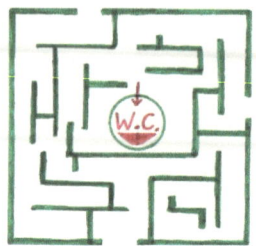

If the chart shows that you have to hold yourself to stop passing urine, perhaps as you get into the house or standing in the queue at the Public Toilets, or that you do start going too early, you have 'urge incontinence'.

Everyone experiences urge incontinence occasionally. However, your bladder to brain to bladder sphincter messages have gone a little awry.

Once your bladder is reasonably full, the message that your bladder sends to the brain is acted on straightaway, without conferring with you to see if it is a convenient time. Alternatively, you may be asking your bladder sphincter to wait, but you then give it the OK before you should do.

Often, the worst time for you is when you are nearly at the loo. Undoing your clothes in the bathroom or putting the key in the front door whilst thinking you are nearly there having been needing to go for a while.

1. Understanding why you have the problem will go a fair way in helping you to solve it. Learn to trick the brain to think of something else until you are actually sitting on the loo. This is easier said than done. It has to be something simple but engrossing, perhaps working out the 13x tables or deciding on the menu for the weekend. Thinking these thoughts until you are actually sitting on the loo will take lots of practice.

2. As with other bladder problems, you may have decreased your intake of fluid to help counter the embarrassing accidents. Your urine will therefore be quite strong and an irritant. Cut down on tea, coffee and alcohol, and make sure you drink at least two litres of fluid a day. This will improve the clarity of messages from your bladder to your brain.

3. PFEs are also necessary to alleviate the pressure on the bladder sphincter.

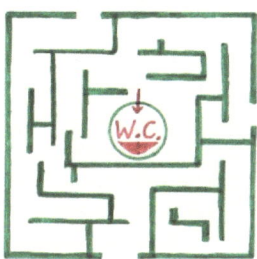

Getting Up at Night to Pass Urine

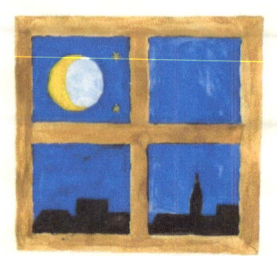

Time	Urine	Damp or change of pad	Reason for Dampness	Other notes
\multicolumn{5}{c}{**A Typical 24-hour Urine Chart When You Have to Get Up at Night**}				
07.30	200mls			Light- coloured urine
09.00	200mls			
11.30	250mls			
13.00	200mls			
15.30	300mls			
18.00	200mls			
23.00	200mls			
01.00	200mls			
03.30	200mls			
Total	1950 mls			

Getting Up at Night to Pass Urine

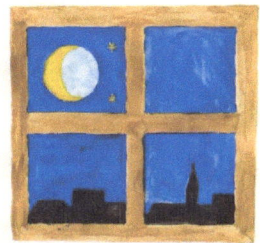

If the chart is showing that you are getting up at night to pas urine this needs to stop. You will find that this is going to persist and increase as your kidneys will produce equal amounts of fluid day and night instead of resting with the rest of the body unless you do something about it.

Kidneys do not go to sleep at night if your body has ingested too much tea, coffee or alcohol. Stress can also keep the body, and kidneys, alert even when we are asleep.

If the urine in the bladder is too concentrated because you have cut down on fluids before going to bed the result will irritate the bladder to think that it needs to empty.

It is normal to wake during the night for a few minutes. When and if you do then you will also need to train yourself to ignore your bladder when you do wake.

1. Refuse tea, coffee and alcohol a few hours before you go to bed.

2. Sleep through the night. There are a variety of things that could help you to sleep through the night. Rather than watching racy television or reading a blood-curdling thriller just before sleep, try some relaxation, perhaps a warm but not hot bath. Relaxation exercises can be done in bed just before sleep.

3. When you do wake up, try to go back to sleep rather than getting up to pass urine. Sometimes you will not go straight back to sleep but resist the temptation to get up and just try to relax.

4. Try not to visit the loo to pass urine the first time you wake. You will not wet the bed in your sleep.

5. Please make sure that you drink at least two litres of fluid daily.

6. Repeat the chart in two weeks' time and you should see that you are sleeping through the night, or at least getting up less often.

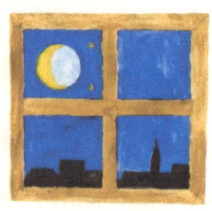

Cystitis

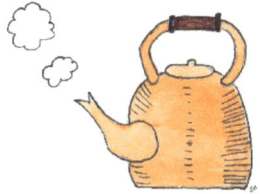

If you have a burning sensation on passing urine, I expect you have cystitis which is a bacterial infection within the bladder. Persistent cystitis is a terribly uncomfortable condition to put up with. Seeing your doctor is a must but after treatment, there are a number of ways to prevent further episodes.

1. Drink a glass of cranberry juice daily. It acts as a natural bladder antibiotic. Drinking at least two litres of fluid daily keeps the urine less concentrated and less of an irritant.

2. Encouraging your bladder to hold a normal amount of urine should help. Please read the chapter on passing urine frequently.

3. And, of course, doing PFEs will support your bladder sphincter. Your sphincter will have been inflamed during your cystitis therefore good pelvic floor muscles will help support the sphincter.

Bladder Problems that Require Medical Attention

There are a few bladder problems that require medical intervention, but often doctors refer patients to surgeons to get a quick-fix for stress incontinence by tightening up the pelvic floor. Surgery may well help short term, but when the pelvic floor once again becomes weak, the incontinence will return. I strongly advise you to follow the advice given in this book for a long-lasting solution to stress incontinence.

However, there are other reasons for medical intervention.

1. If you have been doing your PFEs every day, every hour, and you have not seen any improvement after three months, please visit your doctor for further advice.

2. If you have pain, pass blood or have a burning sensation when passing urine. You may well need a course of antibiotics.

3. If you think that you may have a prolapsed uterus pressing on your bladder.

4. If, after you have passed urine, you feel that your bladder has not completely emptied, your doctor will refer you to a nurse. She can do a simple test to see if there is any residual urine immediately after you have passed urine. This is a very rare condition, but can be significantly improved. The resulting elasticity of the bladder will be poor, rather like a balloon that has been kept inflated, but this elasticity can be regained if the bladder is encouraged to empty each time. The nurse will advise you how to do this.

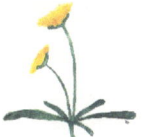

Getting on With Your Life

I hope that you have found this book as clear and concise as I intended. Knowledge and know-how are great tools.

Once you have followed the advice and done your PFEs for a few months you should see a significant improvement but also you will be knowledgeable about your bladder function.

Please keep up those PFEs as they really are the key to keeping good control of your bladder. You should do ten PFEs twice a day, perhaps when you brush your teeth, forever.

Well Done!

There will be many of your friends and colleagues privately, experiencing bladder problems. Perhaps you could spread the word to the one in five women experiencing the assortment of bladder problems and tell them how straightforward it can be to get back in control.

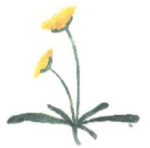

Male Incontinence

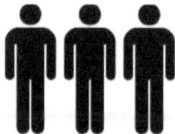

It is rarer for men to have incontinence. They do have pelvic floor muscles, and they do have a bladder to brain to bladder let-down reflex. However, they do not have the trauma of childbirth, which is the primary reason for poor pelvic floor muscle tone.

They can suffer from stress incontinence, urge incontinence, and getting up at night. The advice to treat the problem is the same for men them as for women.

The prostate gland can cause problems for men in later life as it surrounds the urethra. This can cause problems in starting to pass urine, and it may result in a dribbling finish. A visit to the doctor can quickly give a full diagnosis and offer medical treatment if appropriate.

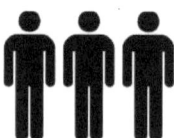

Incontinence of the Bowels

What a tricky one this is, especially with the high incidence of Irritable Bowel Syndrome! It can be so debilitating. However, as this book is for bladder problems, I just feel I cannot ignore the problem completely so here is just a quick resume of the problem.

The food and fluid that we eat and drink are passed straight through our body allowing the absorbtion into the blood stream of the good bits. The resulting waste is then excreted through the anal sphincter.

The process of moving food and fluid from the mouth and through the bowels is called peristalsis. This wave-like motion is set off when we start to eat, and gradually moves the food along through the stomach, small intestine, large intestine and finally the rectum. The waste should wait in the rectum until a convenient time and the brain will then send a message to the anal sphincter to open. If the waste sits in the rectum for too long, it becomes very dry as much of the fluid is absorbed into the body, and constipation can occur.

If the waste rushes through too quickly, insufficient fluid will be absorbed resulting in diarrhea.

The anal sphincter should be able to cope with both diarrhea and constipation. Please seek medical advice if you think that you have sphincter damage.

.

Golden Rules for a Good Bowel

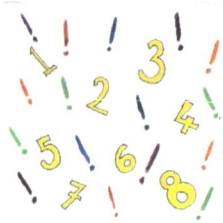

1. Eat 5 portions of vegetables and fruit every day.

2. Drink 2 litres of fluid daily.

3. Take at least twenty minutes' exercise daily.

4. Give yourself time to visit the loo in the morning. You may have been missing the messages saying your rectum is full.

5. Make sure you are not constipated. You can have chronic constipation, rather than incontinence if you have a small bowel movement, often watery, every day. This is actually called constipation with overflow.

6. Seek medical advice if you pass blood, or stools are black (digested blood). NB They may be black if you are on iron supplements.

7. Alleviate stress. This is the most common cause of bowel problems.

Glossary

Bladder
Vessel where urine is stored

Bladder sphincter
The valve or tap which opens to allow urine to be passed

Constipation
The resulting problem when the bowel is overly full with packed waste

Cystitis
Inflammation of the wall of the bladder and sometimes the bladder sphincter. An infection is usually present

Diuretic
A substance that encourages the kdneys to filter more fluid than is normal

Frequency
Passing urine more often than normal

Incontinence
Accidental passing of urine or faeces

Kidney
One of two organs in the body which filter the blood to remove waste products

Micturition
Passing urine

Nocturia
Passing urine at night

Pelvic Floor Muscles
A band of muscles that support the bladder and uterus

Peristalsis
Muscle contractions making a wave-like movement to push food and waste along the bowel

Stools
Waste excreted from the bowel

Stress incontinence
An accidental passing of urine because of extra stress on weak pelvic floor muscles

Ureter
The tube transporting urine from the kidney to the bladder

Urethra
The tube transporting urine from the bladder when you go to the loo

Urge incontinence
An accidental passing of urine due to confused messages from the brain to the bladder sphincter

Urine
Waste product of the blood filtered by the kidneys

Vagina
A tube running parallel to the urethra known as the birth canal, leading to the uterus

24-Hour Urine Chart

Time	Volume	Damp or Change of pads	Reason for Dampness	Other notes
Total For 24 Hours				

24-Hour Urine Chart

Time	Volume	Damp or Change of pads	Reason for Dampness	Other notes
Total For 24 Hours				

24-Hour Urine Chart

Time	Volume	Damp or Change of pads	Reason for Dampness	Other notes
Total For 24 Hours				

24-Hour Urine Chart

Time	Volume	Damp or Change of pads	Reason for Dampness	Other notes
Total For 24 Hours				

24-Hour Urine Chart

Time	Volume	Damp or Change of pads	Reason for Dampness	Other notes
Total For 24 Hours				

Personal Notes